PRELIMINARY INVENTORY OF THE RECORDS OF THE BUREAU OF MEDICINE AND SURGERY

Record Group 52

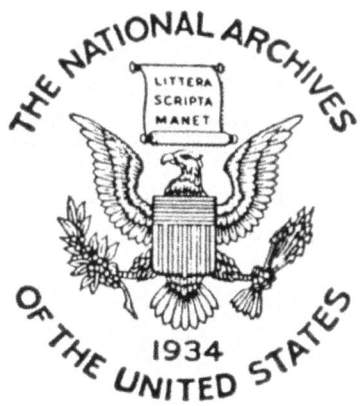

Compiled by
Kenneth F. Bartlett

with
SUPPLEMENT
Compiled by
Harry Schwartz

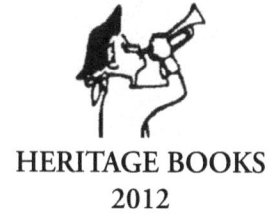

HERITAGE BOOKS
2012

HERITAGE BOOKS
AN IMPRINT OF HERITAGE BOOKS, INC.

Books, CDs, and more—Worldwide

For our listing of thousands of titles see our website
at
www.HeritageBooks.com

A Facsimile Reprint
Published 2012 by
HERITAGE BOOKS, INC.
Publishing Division
100 Railroad Ave. #104
Westminster, Maryland 21157

Originally published

The National Archives
National Archives and Records Service
General Services Administration
Washington: 1948

National Archives Publication No. 48-12

— Publisher's Notice —
In reprints such as this, it is often not possible to remove blemishes from the original. We feel the contents of this book warrant its reissue despite these blemishes and hope you will agree and read it with pleasure.

International Standard Book Numbers
Paperbound: 978-0-7884-3483-9
Clothbound: 978-0-7884-9477-2

THE NATIONAL ARCHIVES

PRELIMINARY INVENTORY OF THE RECORDS
OF THE
BUREAU OF MEDICINE AND SURGERY

Compiled by Kenneth F. Bartlett

Preliminary Inventory No. 6

WASHINGTON : 1948

To make the records in the National Archives more available for use by Government officials, scholars, and other investigators, the Archivist of the United States in February 1941 directed the establishment of a systematic program for the compilation of finding aids. This program includes provision for the compilation of preliminary checklists and preliminary inventories. These preliminary finding aids are prepared without waiting for decisions as to the final arrangement of the records, and in many other respects they are provisional in character. They are intended to be superseded eventually, after the material has been more carefully studied and has been definitively arranged, by final inventories. Other types of finding aids, such as calendars, special lists, and indexes, are compiled from time to time as the need arises and as circumstances permit.

The present work is a preliminary inventory of the materials in Record Group 52, Records of the Bureau of Medicine and Surgery, that had been transferred to the National Archives by April 1948. They amount to about 9,000 cubic feet.

National Archives Publication No. 48-12

CONTENTS

	Page
Introduction	1
Chiefs of the Bureau of Medicine and Surgery, 1842-1948	3
Inventory	5
Headquarters records	5
Correspondence, 1842-1941	5
Medical journals and reports on patients, 1812-1940	9
Medical certificates and casualty lists, 1828-1931	11
Sanitary and other reports, 1907-45	13
Personnel records, 1824-1910	13
Fiscal records, 1893-1926	14
Photographs, 1900-1944	15
Field records	15
Case files for patients at naval hospitals and registers thereto, 1813-1944	15
Records of the Naval Medical School and its predecessors, 1880-1911	16
Other field records, 1859-1920	17

INTRODUCTION

The Bureau of Medicine and Surgery was created by an act of Congress of August 31, 1842, which abolished the Board of Navy Commissioners and established the bureau system in the Navy Department. Of the five bureaus established at that time, the Bureau of Medicine and Surgery is the only one that has been continued to the present day without change in title. The central functions of the Bureau have been formalized and expanded but remain essentially unchanged. They are the care of the sick and injured of the Navy; the administration of naval dispensaries and hospitals; the medical examination of prospective officers and enlisted men and of naval personnel seeking examination or ordered to undergo it for various administrative purposes; and the practice of preventive naval medicine, including inspections of ships and stations to determine the degree of adequacy of food, water supply, arrangements for heat and air, cleanliness, and related factors of health. Research in naval medicine and the specialized instruction of medical officers and selected enlisted men in naval medical practice were conducted informally and individually during the earlier period; in 1939 they culminated in the establishment of what later became the National Naval Medical Center at Bethesda, Md., a group command now consisting of a hospital, medical school, dental school, hospital corps school, medical research institute, and school of hospital administration.

The records of the Bureau of Medicine and Surgery in the National Archives and described in this inventory may be divided into two main parts: Records of the Washington headquarters, 1812-1945, and records of naval medical establishments located in the field, 1813-1944.

The correspondence files of the Bureau are remarkable in that they comprise continuous series of copies of letters sent and of letters received from the establishment of the Bureau to 1941. This circumstance is not characteristic of records of other Navy bureaus and appears to be a result of the long-continued stability of organization of the Bureau. From September 1842 to February 1885 the Bureau employed the copybook system then in vogue in the Navy Department. Under this system letters received were filed in stubbed binders and press copies were made of letters sent. When the course of business permitted, handwritten copies of the press copies of letters sent were made in substantially constructed volumes; these appear to have been regarded as the record copies, although errors in transcription, not found in the facsimile press copies, sometimes occurred. The system also involved keeping registers of letters received and indexes of letters sent.

In February 1885 the docket system of correspondence filing was introduced in the Bureau. Under this system, a serial number was assigned to each letter as it was received. The same number was put on a slip of paper measuring $3\frac{1}{2}$ inches by $8\frac{1}{2}$ inches. The letter was abstracted on the slip, and the two were filed together, except when the letter related to a docket already established. When the letter related to an established docket it was made part of the docket, the abstract slip being filed independently under the number that had been assigned to both the letter and the slip. A note was made on the slip to show where the letter was filed. The file resulting from this system is thus comprised of independently filed abstract slips and of dockets. The slips register the letters received. The dockets consist of abstract slips and of letters received and copies of letters sent folded to the size of the slips. A card index to the system dates from 1896. The press copies in the docket file are duplicated by those in press copybooks from July 1895 to December 1911. After the latter date press copying of letters sent was discontinued in favor of making carbon copies on the typewriter, a machine that had been used in the Bureau since the 1890's.

The docket system was abolished and a series of flat files was established early in 1912 and was continued until 1926. This series is indexed in the card index begun in 1896 and referred to above. Letters received were abstracted on slips as in the docket period; the slips were not filed with the correspondence but were filed together to constitute a register. It is doubtful if all letters received in the latter part of this period were abstracted.

The Secretary of the Navy, on July 5, 1923, directed that the Navy Filing Manual, which was compiled by a board appointed for the purpose, be adopted as a guide for filing throughout the entire naval service exclusive of the Marine Corps. This system employs letters and numerals in combination to produce file symbols of arbitrary subjective significance. Some of the main class symbols, however, may be considered to be abbreviations and others possess independent mnemonic values. The system was introduced in the Bureau of Medicine and Surgery in 1926 when a general correspondence file was established. This file, which has been transferred to the National Archives through 1941, is registered and indexed in a card file.

Many of the headquarters records were prepared in the field and were sent in to headquarters for review and filing. Among such records are the medical journals, amounting to 1,400 kept on board ship, 1813-89 (with gaps especially before 1835), and 321 kept at shore stations, 1812-89. Dr. William P. C. Barton, first Chief of the Bureau, emphasized the importance of keeping medical journals systematically, and most of the journals are for the period after he took office. The "abstracts of patients," 1830-89, likewise were prepared on board ships and at naval hospitals and dispensaries at shore stations to show persons admitted to the sick list and the reasons for such action. The "hospital tickets and case papers," 1825-89, give fuller histories of the cases. Also submitted to headquarters were certificates relating to the medical examination of officers and enlisted men leaving the active naval service, 1842-96, which are in the series entitled "Certificates of Death, Disability, Pension, and Medical Survey" and comprise 129 volumes. Certificates relating to medical examinations made at the time of entrance into the Navy date from 1861 to 1889 and consist of 54 volumes. Other such records include medical histories of naval officers, 1884-99; lists of Navy and Marine Corps dead, 1829-80, with gaps; casualty lists, 1861-70; burial records,

1898-1931; sanitary reports, 1907-43; and reports relating to shipwreck survivors, 1942-45. Also among the headquarters records are personnel records of medical officers and hospital personnel, 1824-1910; fragmentary fiscal records, 1893-1926; and photographs, 1900-1944.

The field records consist largely of case files for patients at 16 naval hospitals and aboard the hospital ship Relief, 1914-39, which are of greater volume than all other records herein described taken together. There are registers of patients at hospitals and dispensaries, 1830-89, with a few as early as 1813 and some as late as 1942 and with some microfilm copies to 1944. Other field records, fragmentary in character, include letters sent by ships' surgeons, 1859-86, records of the Naval Medical School and its predecessors, 1880-1911, and records of the Medical Aide, United States Naval Forces Operating in European Waters, 1918-20.

In this inventory titles have been assigned by the compiler for each entry. Titles in quotation marks are those appearing on the records themselves. Measurements in the entries are in terms of linear feet and inches except for microfilm, which is measured by number of rolls.

Chiefs of the Bureau of Medicine and Surgery, 1842-1948

Surgeon William P. C. Barton, first to hold the office, was commissioned "Chief of the Bureau of Medicine and Surgery," as were his successors until the passage of an act of Congress of March 3, 1871, which provided that the Chief of the Bureau should also hold the title of Surgeon General of the Navy and the relative rank and pay of a commodore. An act of March 3, 1899, gave the Surgeon General the rank of rear admiral, and in 1944 the rank of vice admiral was attached to the office. A list of the Chiefs of the Bureau, with their terms of office, follows:

William P. C. Barton	Sept. 1, 1842-Mar. 31, 1844
Thomas Harris	Apr. 1, 1844-Sept. 30, 1853
William Whelan	Oct. 1, 1853-June 11, 1865
Phineas J. Horwitz	June 12, 1865-June 30, 1869
William M. Wood	July 1, 1869-Oct. 24, 1871
Jonathan M. Foltz	Oct. 25, 1871-June 9, 1872
James C. Palmer	June 10, 1872-July 4, 1873
Joseph Beale	July 5, 1873-Dec. 30, 1876
William Grier	Feb. 2, 1877-Oct. 5, 1878
J. Winthrop Taylor	Oct. 31, 1878-Aug. 19, 1879
Philip S. Wales	Jan. 26, 1880-Jan. 26, 1884
Francis M. Gunnell	Mar. 27, 1884-Mar. 26, 1888
John M. Browne	Apr. 2, 1888-May 9, 1893
James R. Tryon	Sept. 7, 1893-Sept. 7, 1897
William K. Van Reypen	Oct. 22, 1897-Jan. 25, 1902
Presley M. Rixey	Feb. 10, 1902-Feb. 4, 1910
Charles F. Stokes	Feb. 7, 1910-Feb. 10, 1914
William C. Braisted	Feb. 11, 1914-Nov. 29, 1920
Edward R. Stitt	Nov. 30, 1920-Dec. 31, 1928

Charles E. Riggs	Jan. 19, 1929-Mar. 15, 1933
Perceval S. Rossiter	Mar. 16, 1933-Dec. 1, 1938
Ross T. McIntire	Dec. 1, 1938-Dec. 1, 1946
Clifford A. Swanson	Dec. 1, 1946-

RECORDS OF THE BUREAU OF MEDICINE AND SURGERY

HEADQUARTERS RECORDS

Correspondence, 1842-1941

LETTERS SENT ("LETTER BOOK"). Sept. 1842-Feb. 1886. 47 vols. 7 ft., 6 in.

1

Handwritten copies of letters sent by the Chief or Acting Chief of the Bureau, chiefly to medical officers, such as medical directors, surgeons of the fleet, surgeons, and assistant surgeons. Other letters are addressed to commanding officers of stations and squadrons, officials of the Navy Department, naval agents, naval storekeepers, and others. Copies of memoranda issued by the Bureau are included. The letters relate to all business of the Bureau, including the procurement and disposition of medical stores and equipment for ships, dispensaries, and hospitals; medical surveys and pension matters; the appointment of medical officers, surgeon's stewards, apothecaries, and civil employees; admissions to the Government Hospital for the Insane; and the preparation and submission of periodic and special reports. Arranged chronologically. Indexed by name of addressee in front of each volume and in the series described in entries 6 and 8 for periods covered.

LETTERS SENT ("PRESSED LETTERS"). Sept. 1842-June 1864. 28 vols. 5 ft.

2

Press copies that duplicate, in content, the letter books of the above entry for the period covered. A few copies of letters not sent as first written are included, and minor discrepancies are found. The earlier volumes are unlabeled. Arranged chronologically. Indexed in part in the series described in entry 6.

LETTERS RECEIVED ("LETTER BOOK"). Sept. 1842-Dec. 1856. 114 vols. 22 ft.

3

Letters received relating to the same matters dealt with in the letters sent described in entry 1. The volumes are numbered serially for each year; on the backstrip of each volume are stamped the year, the serial number thereunder, and the class or classes of sender. Arranged by year, thereunder by class of sender ("Surgeons and Assistant Surgeons," "Officers Not Medical," "Secretary of the Navy and Chiefs of Bureaus," "Naval Agents," "Naval Storekeepers," and "Miscellaneous"), thereunder chronologically. Indexed by name or office of sender in front of each volume.

LETTERS SENT ("MISCELLANEOUS," "LETTERS FROM ALL SOURCES"). Apr.-May 1866, Oct. 1878-Apr. 1879, Jan.-Apr. 1880, Dec. 1883-Aug. 1884, June-Dec. 1887, Mar.-Apr. 1888. 8 vols. 1 ft.

4

A fragmentary series of press copies. No speciality of subject is apparent, and the letters were sent over the Bureau Chief's signature

5

in the usual manner. The two volumes stamped "Letters from All Sources" appear to be mislabeled. Arranged chronologically. Indexed in part in series described in entry 8.

LETTERS SENT TO THE NAVAL LABORATORY, NEW YORK ("LETTER BOOK. DIRECTOR OF THE LABORATORY, NO. 2"). Jan. 1865-July 1870. 1 vol. 2 1/2 in. **5**
Copies of letters addressed to the Director, Naval Laboratory, New York, relating mainly to the distribution of medical stores to ships and stations. The Laboratory served as a medical storehouse and the Director was a medical officer. Other letters relate to the examination of applicants for appointments as medical officers, medical and sanitary inspections of vessels, and kindred matters. Arranged chronologically. Name and subject index in front of volume.

INDEXES TO LETTERS SENT ("KEY TO LETTERS NO. 5" AND "INDEX TO LETTERS, 1875-1877"). May 1848-Dec. 1849, Dec. 1875-Mar. 1877. 2 vols. 5 in. **6**
Indexes to series described in entries 1 and 2 for periods covered. Gives name and station of writer and date and subject of letter. Arranged by initial letter of name of addressee, thereunder chronologically.

LETTERS RECEIVED ("LETTERS FROM ALL SOURCES"). Jan. 1857-Feb. 1885. 298 vols. 59 ft. **7**
A general file of letters received, which differs from the earlier file described in entry 3 in that filing by class of sender is discontinued. Arranged in a single chronological series, the year and serial number thereunder being stamped on the backs of the volumes. Indexed by name or office of sender in front of each volume and registered in part in the series described in entries 8 and 9.

REGISTER AND INDEX TO CORRESPONDENCE. Mar. 1882-Feb. 1885. 1 vol. 3 in. **8**
Register of letters received (entry 7) and index to some of the letters sent described in entries 1 and 4. Gives name of writer or addressee, date and purport of letter, and action taken in response thereto (for letters received). Arranged in two parts, chronologically for letters received and alphabetically, thereunder chronologically, for letters sent.

REGISTERS OF LETTERS RECEIVED ("REGISTER OF LETTERS" AND "LETTERS RECEIVED"). Jan. 1860-Oct. 1863, Jan. 1865-Dec. 1868, July 1870-Sept. 1878, July 1886-Dec. 1887. 11 vols. 1 ft., 10 in. **9**
Gives date of receipt of letter and file number assigned; author, date, and purport of letter; action taken. Register in part for the series described in entries 7 and 11. Arranged chronologically, thereunder numerically.

LETTERS SENT. July 1895-Dec. 1911. 97 vols. 31 ft., 6 in. **10**
Press copies that appear to duplicate the press copies of letters sent found in the general correspondence file (entry 11). The year,

month or months, and serial numbers of the letters contained are stamped on the backs of most of the volumes. Arranged numerically and therefore in approximate chronological order. Indexed in part in the series described in entry 13.

GENERAL CORRESPONDENCE. Feb. 1885-Apr. 1912. Folded dockets, 3 1/2" x 8 1/2". 445 ft.   11

    Letters received, press copies of letters sent, and abstract slips of letters received. Memoranda and reports are included, but special forms of reports, such as certificates of death, disability, pension, and medical survey, are filed separately (see entry 31). Duplicates of press copies of letters sent before January 1912 are found in the volumes described in entry 10. Other duplicates, for parts of 1887 and 1888, are found in the series described in entry 4. The file contains handwritten copies of despatches and other items apparently deemed unsuitable for press copying. The docket system of filing correspondence is explained on page 1.

    The docketed general correspondence files are arranged numerically as follows: 1A to 5773A (Mar. 1885-June 1886), 2B to 4439B (July 1886-Dec. 1887), 2A to 3605A (Jan.-Dec. 1888), 6 to 3107 (1889), 1 to 1887 (1890), 1 to 1898 (1891), 1 to 1668 (1892), 1 to 3735 (1893), and 1 to 124676 (1894-Apr. 1912). Registered in the series described in entry 9, July 1886-Dec. 1887, thereafter on the abstract slips in the files; indexed in the series described in entry 13 from 1896 on.

GENERAL CORRESPONDENCE. Mar. 1912-Dec. 1925. 142 ft.   12

    Letters received and copies of letters sent relating to all the business of the Bureau, including health and sanitary conditions, the disposition of the remains of the dead, the establishment and administration of naval hospitals and dispensaries, the development of the Naval Dental Corps, and aviation and submarine medicine. A few letters dated prior to March 1912 and a special file (F-124677-0) consisting mainly of letters from the Graves Registration Service are found at the beginning of the file; subsequent folders are numbered from 124677 to 132699. Arranged numerically. Indexed in the series described in entry 13. Letters received registered in the series described in entry 14.

INDEX TO GENERAL CORRESPONDENCE. 1896-Dec. 1925. Cards, 3" x 5". 8 ft.
                                                                                                                                                                  13

    Index by subject and facility (for example, Norfolk, Va., Hospital) to the series described in entries 11-13. Arranged alphabetically, thereunder chronologically.

REGISTER OF LETTERS RECEIVED. Mar. 1912-Dec. 1925. Slips, 3" x 8". 5 ft.   14

    Abstract slips numbered from 124677 to 132699, similar in form to those described in entry 11 and covering letters received described in entry 12. Beginning in March 1912 correspondence was filed flat and abstract slips were filed separately. Most of the slips, particularly from 1916 to 1920, contain abstracts of letters from reserve medical and dental officers and prospective officers. Arranged numerically.

GENERAL CORRESPONDENCE. Jan. 1926-Dec. 1941. 75 ft., 6 in.   15
    Letters received, copies of letters sent, reports, and memoranda relating to the administration of the Bureau and referring to such matters as the creation of mobile base hospitals, the comprehensive use of X-ray techniques in the control of tuberculosis, the use of barbiturates, sulfonamides, and blood plasma, and industrial hygiene in navy yards. Arranged according to Navy Filing Manual designations. Indexed in the series described in entry 16.

INDEX TO GENERAL CORRESPONDENCE. Jan. 1926-Dec. 1941. Cards, 7 1/4" x 9 1/4". 8 ft., 6 in.   16
    Combined subject index and register for the series described in entry 15. Letters are registered under name of sender or addressee and indexed under selected subject headings. Not all letters are indexed. Arranged alphabetically, thereunder chronologically.

SECRET AND CONFIDENTIAL CORRESPONDENCE. Aug. 1920-Dec. 1941. 6 ft. 3 in.   17
    Letters, reports, and memoranda concerning war plans, psychological and physiological experimentation and investigation, emergency requirements of medical personnel, medicines, hospital and dispensary facilities, and related matters. These files were received from the Planning Division, which is charged with the control of classified files. There are only a few folders for the years prior to 1931 and none for the year 1921. Arranged chronologically. Registered in the series described in entry 18.

REGISTER OF SECRET AND CONFIDENTIAL CORRESPONDENCE. Aug. 1920-Dec. 1941. 1 roll of microfilm and 2 in. of photographic prints, 8" x 8".   18
    One roll of 16 mm. negative microfilm copies of 7 1/4" x 9 1/4" cards, upon which is registered the series described in entry 17, and positive photographic prints of the same. The original cards have been retained by the Bureau. Arranged chronologically.

CORRESPONDENCE RELATING TO THE HOSPITAL CORPS TRAINING SCHOOL. Sept. 1902-Feb. 1911. 2 1/2 in.   19
    Letters received and copies of letters sent, including letters from commanding officers of naval hospitals recommending apprentices for training at the School, letters from the commanding officer of the School, and copies of letters sent to the Bureau of Navigation recommending the assignment of the graduates of the School. The School, established at the Norfolk Naval Hospital in 1902, was transferred to the Washington Naval Hospital in 1907 and continued in existence until the founding of the Naval Medical School in 1911.

LETTERS SENT BY THE SUPERINTENDENT OF THE NURSE CORPS. Aug. 1909-Dec. 1911. 3 vols. 4 in.   20
    Press copies of letters addressed chiefly to members and prospective members of the Nurse Corps. The first volume is composed chiefly of letters marked "Personal" and "Semi-official," Aug. 25, 1909-Aug. 2, 1911; a few letters, Oct. 24-Dec. 22, 1911, are not so marked and are

in standard naval form. Letters in another volume, Nov. 21-Dec. 29, 1911, and in one marked "No. 3," Aug. 30, 1910-May 20, 1911, relate mainly to examinations, qualifications, appointments, discharges, and orders. The three volumes appear to represent fragments of at least two original series. Arranged chronologically. Indexed in front of each volume by name of addressee.

Medical Journals and Reports on Patients, 1812-1940

MEDICAL JOURNALS OF SHORE STATIONS. 1812-89. 321 vols. 50 ft.   **21**
    Consists of journals kept at (1) the New York, Portsmouth (N. H.), and Washington Marine Barracks; (2) at the Naval Academy; (3) at the Washington Naval Dispensary; (4) at the Bella Vista (Peru), Chelsea (Mass.), Mare Island (Calif.), Memphis (Tenn.), Mound City (Ill.), New Orleans, New York, Norfolk (Va.), Pensacola (Fla.), Philadelphia, Pilot Town (La.), Portsmouth, St. Helena Island (S. C.), San Jose (Calif.), and Washington Naval Hospitals; (5) at the Baltimore, Bay Point (Maine), Mound City, New London (Conn.), Pensacola, and Port Royal (S. C.) Naval Stations; (6) at the Newport (R. I.) Naval Torpedo Station; and (7) at the Boston, Mare Island, New York, Norfolk, Philadelphia, Portsmouth, and Washington Navy Yards. Includes also six volumes kept at New York, Portsmouth, and Washington labeled "Special Duty."
    The journals vary considerably in style and content, particularly before 1867, when the Bureau of Medicine and Surgery ordered a standard mode of keeping medical journals throughout the Navy. Some of the journals kept before that date have brief entries only; others are more fully descriptive of patients, diagnoses, and treatments. Fatal illnesses are usually described in greater detail.
    From 1867 on, some or all of the following data are found: name of person admitted to the sick list, rate or rank, age, nativity, ship or station of transfer, diagnosis, and treatment; number of persons admitted, number discharged, number deceased, number transferred, and total number on sick list; date of entry; and name and rank of medical officer signing the journal. Exact dosages of medicines prescribed are usually indicated, although general prescriptions such as "ale, wine, and a good diet" are sometimes found. The journals are arranged by type of station (for example, marine barracks or navy yards), thereunder alphabetically by name of city or other location. Indexed in part in the series described in entry 26; individual patients indexed in some volumes.

MEDICAL JOURNALS OF SHIPS. 1813-89. 1,400 vols. 195 ft.   **22**
    These journals are similar to those described in entry 21 and were kept on shipboard by medical officers. There are infrequent comments on the condition of the ship and her crew following a battle or a heavy sea. This is an incomplete series with gaps in coverage that are not self-explanatory. For example, the earliest journal is that of the USS Constitution and dates from March 31, 1813, to October 3, 1813; the next journal in chronological sequence for that ship begins March 13,

1835. These gaps are mainly in the period prior to 1835. Some volumes contain journals of two or more ships.

The journals are arranged in approximate alphabetical order by name of ship, thereunder chronologically. Indexed in part in the series described in entry 26; individual patients indexed in some volumes.

MEDICAL JOURNALS OF EXPEDITIONS. Mar. 1872-May 1885. 3 vols. 4 in. 23

Consists of medical journals of the Greely Relief Expedition (Apr.-Nov. 1884), the Nicaragua Surveying Expedition (Mar. 1872-June 1873), and the Panama Surveying Expedition (Apr. 1884-May 1885). Individual patients indexed in volumes.

"ABSTRACTS OF PATIENTS." 1830-89. 96 vols. 16 ft., 6 in. 24

Lists prepared periodically by field activities and submitted to the Bureau. They show persons admitted to the sick list on board ships and at naval hospitals and dispensaries at shore stations, usually giving for each patient his name, rate or rank, age, place of birth, date of admission, disease or injury, date and manner of discharge, origin of disability in terms of duty status (in line of duty, not in line of duty, or no evidence), and remarks of medical officer (such as "Exposure to cold and wet").

The earliest abstract relates to the USS America. The abstracts are arranged as follows: By name of ship, 1835-Dec. 1873; by location of shore station, 1830-Dec. 1873, and 1876; by year for ships, 1874-80; by year for shore stations, 1874-75, 1877-80; in one chronological series for both ships and stations, 1881-89. Minor exceptions exist. Secondary alphabetical arrangements are found under the chronological arrangements. The names of ships usually appear on the backstrips of the volumes relating to them. Individual entries of patients' names on the lists are usually arranged by initial letter.

"HOSPITAL TICKETS AND CASE PAPERS." 1825-89. 274 vols. 52 ft., 8 in. 25

"Hospital tickets" are letters (usually standard form G), addressed to medical officers in charge of naval hospitals requesting them to receive patients being transferred from ships or stations for hospital treatment. They are sent over the signatures of medical and other officers and usually contain the following information about the patient: name, rate or rank, age, nativity, date and place of shipping aboard, medical history, present diagnosis, and list of clothing.

The "case papers" (usually standard form H), are bound with the hospital tickets to which they relate and show the hospital treatment and eventual disposition of the cases. There are hospital tickets and case papers for the following hospitals: Annapolis, Beaufort (N. C.), Chelsea (Mass.), Hong Kong, Key West, Mare Island (Calif.), Memphis (Pinkney Hospital), Mound City (Ill.), New Orleans, New York, Norfolk, Pensacola (Fla.), Philadelphia, Pilot Town (La.) [bound with Beaufort], Portsmouth (N. H.), Port Royal (S. C.), Washington, and Yokohama. An anomalous volume relates to the Mississippi Squadron, 1862-64. Arranged alphabetically by location of hospital. Indexed by name of patient in front of each volume.

LISTS OF MEDICAL RECORDS. 1613-1912. 2 vols. 3 in.   26
    Lists of medical journals, abstracts of patients, and hospital tickets and case papers received from ships and stations by the Bureau. Partial index to entries 21-25. Arranged alphabetically by name of ship and location of shore station, thereunder chronologically.

REPORTS OF PATIENTS. 1917, 1919, 1928-40. Slips, 3" x 5". 498 ft.   27
    Slips (forms F and FA) prepared by ship or station on which patient was stationed at time of illness. Data entered on cards include patient's name, date and place of birth, length of service, rank or rate, diagnosis, manner of admission and discharge, and place of admission. If the patient had been injured, the cause was given. Arranged by year, thereunder by name of patient.

LISTS OF PERSONS INVALIDED FROM THE SERVICE. 1918-39. Slips, 3" x 5". 25 ft., 4 in.   28
    Copies of FA forms (described above) arranged to form lists of naval personnel invalided from the service. Arranged by year, thereunder by name of patient.

ABSTRACTS OF SICK REPORTS. Oct. 1851-June 1880. 4 vols. 9 in.   29
    Abstracts of reports made by ships and stations showing number of admissions, discharges, and deaths. Parallel columns give summaries of expenses for provisions, groceries, medicines, and incidentals and computations of the average number of patients and average cost per man daily. Includes also a volume entitled "Form K, Hospitals, Ships and Stations for the Year 1869," which consists of summary sick reports.

Medical Certificates and Casualty Lists, 1828-1931

REPORTS OF DISEASES AND DEATHS ("MISCELLANEOUS REPORTS: DEATHS, DISCHARGES, DISEASES, PATIENTS"). July 1828-Dec. 1846. 1 vol. 2 1/2 in.   30
    Consists of (1) a letter of July 7, 1828, addressed to Secretary of the Navy Samuel L. Southard by Thomas Harris, then Surgeon at the Philadelphia Hospital and later Chief of the Bureau of Medicine and Surgery, reporting that certain medical officers are receiving instruction under him; (2) monthly reports of deaths on board ships of the Navy; and (3) quarterly reports of the sick on ships and at naval hospitals and navy yards. Arranged chronologically.

CERTIFICATES OF DEATH, DISABILITY, PENSION, AND MEDICAL SURVEY. June 1842-Jan. 1896. 137 vols. 23 ft., 6 in.   31
    Letters and certificates relating to medical examinations of officers and enlisted men of the Navy and the Marine Corps, consisting of a single chronological series of 129 volumes, June 1842-Jan. 1896, and of the following volumes: (1) "Certificates of Disability, Supplementary," 1852-62; (2) "Certificates of Death," 1852-62; (3) "Certificates of Ordinary Disability and Certificates of Death, Nov. 1862-Dec. 1867;" (4) "Certificates of Death, Navy Yard, Boston, Mass., and USS Hendrick Hudson, 1864-1873;" (5) "Certificates of Death, Naval Hospital,

Norfolk, Va., Aug. 1874-Nov. 1879;" (6) "Miscellaneous Medical Surveys, Mar. 1859-Oct. 1877;" (7) "Reports of Surveys (copies), Naval Hospital, New York, N. Y., Jan. 1866-Jan. 1868;" and (8) "Reports of Surveys, Certificates of Death and Ordinary Disability, Jan. 9, 1868 [-Dec. 20, 1877], Naval Hospital, New York." Arranged chronologically, except for item 7, which is arranged alphabetically by name of person examined. Indexed in fronts of some volumes; the 129-volume series is indexed in the series described in the following entry.

INDEX TO CERTIFICATES OF DEATH, DISABILITY, PENSION, AND MEDICAL SURVEY. June 1842-Jan. 1896. 2 vols. 5 in.   32
    Index to the series of 129 volumes described in the above entry. References are to volume and page by number. Arranged alphabetically by name of person examined.

CERTIFICATES OF PHYSICAL EXAMINATION. 1861-89. 54 vols. 10 ft.   33
    Certificates executed by medical examiners at naval and marine recruiting and other centers at Baltimore, Boston, Buffalo, Cleveland, Erie, Mound City (Ill.), New Orleans, New York, and Washington. Included are (1) a volume entitled "Record of Physical Examination of Candidates for Admission Into the Regular Navy Who Appeared Before the Naval Board Convened at Hartford, Conn., Sept. 5, 1866;" (2) 2 volumes relating to engineers, paymasters, gunners, boatswains, carpenters, and mates examined at the New York Navy Yard; and (3) 11 volumes entitled "List of Persons Examined for the Naval Service." Arranged alphabetically by city, thereunder chronologically, except that item 3 is arranged chronologically.

OFFICERS' MEDICAL RECORDS ("RECORDS FOR RETIREMENT" AND "RECORDS FOR PROMOTION"). Feb. 1884-Mar. 1899. 2 vols. 6 in.   34
    Press copies of individual medical histories of commissioned and warrant officers, compiled from medical journals, hospital papers, and related records for the use of retiring boards in the case of the first volume (Feb. 1884-Feb. 1899) and for the use of examining boards for promotion in the case of the second volume (June 1890-Mar. 1899). The histories are in the form of letters sent over the signature of the Surgeon General or the Acting Chief of the Bureau. Arranged chronologically. Indexed in each volume.

DEATH LISTS. 1829-43, 1858-65, 1868-80. 5 vols. 6 in.   35
    Lists of Navy and Marine Corps dead, usually giving name, rate or rank, date and cause of death, and a statement as to whether or not the disease or injury originated in the line of duty. Arranged chronologically, sometimes under the name of the ship or station; but the volume for 1858-65 is arranged by name of the deceased.

CASUALTY LISTS. 1861-70, 1917. 2 vols. and 1 portfolio. 6 in.   36
    Consists of (1) a volume entitled "Casualties in the U. S. Navy, Apr. 1861 to July 1865;" (2) a supplemental volume, "Casualties, Apr. 1862 to July 1870;" and (3) lists of sick and wounded of the Fifth Regiment, Marine Corps, Second Division, American Expeditionary Forces,

France, July to December 1917. Items 1 and 3 arranged chronologically and item 2 arranged alphabetically. Item 1 indexed by name in the front of the volume.

BURIAL RECORDS. 1898-1931. 26 vols. 3 ft., 6 in. 37
Lists kept on hospital ships and at naval hospitals and other stations, relating to the disposition of the remains of the dead. Arranged by name of ship or station, thereunder chronologically.

Sanitary and Other Reports, 1907-45

ANNUAL SANITARY REPORTS. 1907-16, 1919-43. 95 ft. 38
Reports submitted by medical officers of ships, naval stations, and naval hospitals. They relate to conditions of ships, buildings, and grounds with reference to cleanliness, ventilation, water supply, drainage, heating, disposition of the dead, and like subjects. Arranged by year, thereunder alphabetically.

MONTHLY SANITARY REPORTS. 1926-43. 40 ft. 39
Reports of sanitary conditions at shore activities in the field, including reports of overseas activities. Monthly sanitary reports for 1907-25 are filed in the general correspondence files (entries 11 and 12) and indexed in the series described in entry 13. Arranged by year, thereunder numerically by naval district, thereunder alphabetically by location of activity.

REPORTS RELATING TO RESCUED SURVIVORS OF WRECKED SHIPS AND AIRCRAFT. 1942-45. 1 ft., 3 in. 40
A Bureau letter dated April 14, 1942, directed that reports in prescribed form should be made by medical officers when survivors of wrecked, sunken, or abandoned ships or aircraft were rescued by Navy ships. The letters comprising this file were written mainly in response to the directive and concern the nature of injuries and illnesses sustained, duration of exposure, condition and treatment of the rescued, and recommendations. Most of the reports were formerly classified "Secret" but are now declassified. Arranged in folders bearing the following labels: Aircraft, Belgian Vessel, H. M. S. British, French Navy Tanker, German Vessels, Japanese, Coast, S. S. [Merchant] Vessels, U. S. A. T. [Army Transport], U. S. S. [Navy] Vessels, and Misc., Name Not Given or Vessels Sunk Unknown.

Personnel Records, 1824-1910

LIST OF MEDICAL OFFICERS. 1824-73. 1 vol. 2 in. 41
List of medical officers on duty on ships and at stations, giving for each officer dates of attachment and detachment and, for the earlier period, computations of his tour of duty in years, months, and days. Arranged by name of ship or station, thereunder chronologically. Indexed by name of ship or station in front of volume.

APPLICATIONS AND ORDERS OF MEDICAL OFFICERS ("ORDERS" AND "APPLICATIONS AND ORDERS"). Aug. 1844-Dec. 1857, July 1861-Feb. 1895. 12 vols. 2 ft. 42

The earlier volumes, stamped "Orders," contain copies of orders addressed to individual medical officers; the later "Applications and Orders" consist of copies of orders and copies of letters received from officers requesting assignments to duty, usually at specified stations. The volumes are numbered serially from 1 to 13, with volume 6 missing. Arranged chronologically. Indexed by name in front of each volume.

STATEMENTS OF SERVICE OF MEDICAL OFFICERS ("ORDERS OF MEDICAL OFFICERS"). 1842-73. 1 vol. 2 in. 43

Summary statements regarding appointment, orders to duty, reporting for duty, promotion, retirement, resignation, dismissal, and death for officers active in the first three decades of the Bureau's existence. Arranged chronologically. Indexed in front of volume.

STATEMENTS OF SERVICE OF ACTING MEDICAL OFFICERS ("ACTING MEDICAL OFFICERS"). 1860-70. 1 vol. 2 in. 44

Summaries of service of acting officers, mainly for the period 1861-65. Arranged alphabetically by name of officer. Indexed in front of volume.

APPOINTMENT PAPERS OF SURGEON'S STEWARDS, APOTHECARIES, AND NURSES ("SURGEON'S STEWARDS"). 1861-84. 6 vols. 1 ft., 2 in. 45

Articles of agreement and oaths of allegiance executed by surgeon's stewards, apothecaries, and nurses upon entrance into the Navy and related papers. Arranged chronologically. Indexed in the front of each volume and in lists accompanying the records. These papers are continued in entry 46.

CASE FILES FOR HOSPITAL PERSONNEL ("PERSONNEL JACKETS"). 1884-1910. 20 ft. 46

Applications for enlistment, examination reports, orders, proficiency reports, and related records. Arranged alphabetically.

Fiscal Records, 1893-1926

JOURNAL OF EXPENDITURES AND RECEIPTS ("DAY BOOK NO. 11"). Feb. 1893-Jan. 1898. 1 vol. 2 1/2 in. 47

A journal listing debits and credits, balanced monthly to show unexpended moneys in the several funds appropriated for the expenses of activities under the cognizance of the Bureau. Arranged chronologically.

JOURNAL OF EXPENDITURES ("DAY BOOK"). 1922-26. 6 vols. 1 ft., 8 in. 48
Shows moneys expended from the several appropriations for activities under the cognizance of the Bureau on ships, in naval hospitals, and elsewhere. Arranged alphabetically.

14

Photographs, 1900-1944

PHOTOGRAPHS. 1900-1944. 13 in. of prints and negatives and 2 in. of
lantern slides. 49
  Photographic prints showing the Washington Naval Hospital, 1900, the Norfolk Naval Hospital, 1918-19, and the Hospital Corps Training School at these hospitals, 1903-11; lantern slides showing vapor clouds, gas shells, gas masks, and treatment of gassed soldiers, 1918-19; and photographic prints and negatives made by field medical photographic units of the Bureau on Utah Beach, Normandy, and in England to illustrate the care of the wounded, 1944.

FIELD RECORDS

Case Files for Patients at Naval Hospitals and Registers Thereto 1813-1944

CASE FILES FOR PATIENTS ("PATIENTS' JACKETS"). 1914-39. Envelopes and
folders, various sizes. 9,153 ft. 50
  Hospital record jackets for patients at the following hospitals: Annapolis (1920-39), Brooklyn (1921-39), Chelsea, Mass. (1919-39), Charleston (1920-39), Great Lakes (1921-39), Mare Island, Calif. (1918-39), Newport, R. I. (1920-38), Norfolk (Portsmouth, Va., 1918-39), Parris Island, S. C. (1918-39), Pearl Harbor (1921-39), Philadelphia (1917-39), Portsmouth, N. H. (1918-38), Puget Sound (Bremerton, Wash., 1919-39), Quantico, Va. (1922-39), San Diego (1919-39), and Washington (1914-39; the Washington Naval Hospital became a part of the Naval Medical Center, Washington, upon its establishment in 1935). Includes also jackets for patients on board the hospital ship Relief (1921-39). The dates are dates of admission to the hospitals; some of the records are dated as late as 1945.
  The jackets contain clinical records and correspondence relating to diagnoses, treatments, admissions, and discharges. The clinical records include fever charts, electrocardiographs, and similar papers. Included in the files from some hospitals are personnel jackets for hospital corpsmen, apparently filed with patients' jackets as a matter of convenience. Arranged by serial case numbers in one or more series for each hospital. Registered in part in series described in entries 51 and 52.

REGISTERS OF PATIENTS. 1813-1942. 109 vols. and 8 envelopes of photostats. 22 ft., 8 in. 51
  Registers of patients on ships and at Navy and Marine Corps hospitals and dispensaries, varying in details of form and content with the periods covered but usually giving for each patient his name, rate or rank, age, birthplace, and disease or injury and the disposition of the case (that is, by discharge to duty or to another hospital, by discharge for disability, or by death). Case numbers for individual patients are found in the more recent volumes, which serve as finding aids to some of the patients' jackets described in entry 50. The only registers dating later than 1940 are photostat copies of registers for

15

the Bremerton Naval Hospital, which extend into 1942. Included are registers for the hospital ships Comfort (1918-21) and Mercy (1918-29).

Registers for shore stations include those for hospitals at the following locations in foreign countries or territories or possessions of the United States: Brest, France (1917-19), Leith, Scotland (1918-19), London (1918-19), Lorient, France (1918-19), Olongapo, P. I. (1911-17), Pearl Harbor (1917-40), Port-au-Prince, Haiti (1920-34), Ponta Delgada, Azores (1918-19), St. Thomas, V. I. (1917-31), San Juan, P. R. (1899-1911), Sitka, Alaska (1894-1911), Strathpeffer, Scotland (1918-19), and Tientsin, China (1927-29).

Arranged by name of ship or by name or location of shore station, thereunder chronologically. Entries for individual patients are usually arranged by initial letter of name. Some volumes are indexed in front or back.

MICROFILM COPIES OF REGISTERS OF PATIENTS. 1915-44. 48 rolls. 52

Copies of registers kept at the following naval hospitals: Annapolis (1917-40), Brooklyn (1920-39), Charleston (1917-42), Chelsea, Mass. (1919-39), Great Lakes Naval Training Station, Ill. (1917-40), Newport, R. I. (1920-40), Parris Island, S. C. (1931-41), Philadelphia (1915-40), Portsmouth, N. H. (1917-44), and Quantico, Va. (1933-41). Serve as finding aids to some of the patients' jackets described in entry 50. Arranged alphabetically by hospital, thereunder chronologically.

Records of the Naval Medical School and Its Predecessors
1880-1911

An Experimental Laboratory was established in the Surgeon General's Office in 1879. In 1882 a building at or near 18th and G Streets, N. W., Washington, was rented by the Bureau of Medicine and Surgery to provide quarters for a new establishment designated the United States Naval Museum of Hygiene, of which the Laboratory was made a part. In 1894 the Museum moved to the old Naval Observatory Building at the foot of 24th Street, N. W., which had been vacated in favor of the new Observatory Building in Georgetown Heights, D. C.

The Museum became the United States Naval Museum of Hygiene and Medical School in 1902. The School was a revival of an earlier school for medical officers that had been located at New York as part of the former United States Naval Laboratory and Department of Instruction but that had been discontinued during the Spanish-American War. The Museum was discontinued in 1905 and its exhibits were transferred to the National Museum. The work of the Hospital Corps Training School, which had been established at the Norfolk Naval Hospital in 1902 and had been transferred to the Washington Naval Hospital in 1907, was taken over by the Naval Medical School in 1911.

LETTERS SENT. June 1880-Apr. 1909. 15 vols. 2 ft., 7 in. 53

Press copies of letters sent by the Experimental Laboratory (Mar. 1880-Apr. 1882), the Naval Museum of Hygiene (Apr. 1882-Oct. 1902), the combined Museum of Hygiene and Medical School (Oct. 1902-May 1905), and the Naval Medical School (May 1905-Apr. 1909). The Experimental Laboratory sent some letters under its own letterhead after becoming part of the Museum of Hygiene; the last of these is dated December 8, 1882. Includes one volume of copies of letters sent to the Bureau of Medicine and Surgery exclusively (Sept. 1893-June 1902). Arranged chronologically. Some volumes are indexed in front by name of addressee.

LETTERS RECEIVED. Mar. 1880-Sept. 1911. 15 vols. 4 ft., 5 in. 54
    A general file of letters received, corresponding to the letters sent described in entry 54. Arranged chronologically. Some volumes are indexed in front or back.

LETTERS RECEIVED RELATING TO MICROSCOPES. Sept. 1883-July 1897. 1 vol. 3 in. 55
    Letters received by the Museum of Hygiene from medical and other officers on ships and at stations, relating to the distribution, maintenance, and repair of microscopes and accessories used by medical officers. Includes also a press copy of a special report on the condition of microscopes examined by Medical Inspector J. C. Wise, which was sent to the Bureau of Medicine and Surgery with a letter of November 9, 1896. Arranged chronologically.

ORDERS AND NOTICES OF THE MEDICAL SCHOOL. Aug. 1905-Mar. 1909. 1 vol. 1 1/4 in. 56
    Press copies of circular orders and notices issued by the medical officer in command of the School and relating to the academic schedule, uniform regulations, rules for student officers, and the administration of the School. Includes also a few copies of letters sent. Arranged chronologically. Indexed by subject in front of volume.

CERTIFICATES OF PROFICIENCY GRANTED BY THE HOSPITAL CORPS TRAINING SCHOOL. Dec. 1902-May 1907. 2 vols. 3 1/2 in. 57
    Executed copies of a standard form giving for each student graduated from the Hospital Corps Training School at the Norfolk Naval Hospital his name, rate, date and place of birth, date and place of enlistment, dates of entrance and graduation, and marks for the following subjects: Discipline and drill, nursing, anatomy and physiology, bandaging, aptitude, first aid, hygiene, materia medica, pharmacy, clerical work, and conduct. Correspondence relating to the School is described in entry 19.

Other Field Records, 1859-1920

LETTERS SENT BY SHIPS' SURGEONS ("LETTER BOOK"). 1859-86. 3 vols. 4 in. 58
    Copies of letters sent by surgeons aboard the following ships: USS Portsmouth (Apr. 1859-Sept. 1861), USS Potomac (Jan. 1875-Jan. 1877), USS Constitution (Jan. 1877-Sept. 1881), and USS Kearsarge (Nov. 1879-Oct. 1886). Letters of the Potomac and the Constitution are bound together. Included are copies of quarterly sick reports. Arranged by ship, thereunder chronologically.

CORRESPONDENCE OF THE MEDICAL AIDE, UNITED STATES NAVAL FORCES OPERATING IN EUROPEAN WATERS. 1918-20. 3 ft., 9 in. 59

Consists of (1) an apparently fragmentary series of letters received and copies of letters sent, including requisitions and reports on standard forms; and (2) copies of letters and dispatches originating in the London headquarters of the Commander of the United States Naval Forces Operating in European Waters and relating to deaths of enlisted men in Europe and to the disposition of their bodies and personal effects. Included are reports received from subordinate commanders and correspondence with the Navy Department in Washington. Arranged alphabetically by subject (item 1) and by name of deceased (item 2), except that item 2 begins with a chronological file, Apr. 1918-Jan. 1919.

HM-48

GENERAL SERVICES ADMINISTRATION
NATIONAL ARCHIVES AND RECORDS SERVICE
THE NATIONAL ARCHIVES

Supplement to Preliminary Inventory No. 6

Records of the
Bureau of Medicine and Surgery

(Record Group 52)

Compiled by

Harry Schwartz

1965

This supplement has been reproduced in this form by the Office of Military Archives in order to make it readily available for staff use. It has not been distributed as a National Archives publication.

CONTENTS

	Page
Introduction	1
Inventory	
Headquarters records	3
Correspondence, 1842-1951	3
Medical journals and reports on patients, 1812-1940	3
Medical certificates and casualty lists, 1828-1939	3
Sanitary and other reports, 1907-45	3
Personnel records, 1824-1930	3
Fiscal records, 1854-1926	4
Records relating to the history of naval medicine, 1775-1946	4
Records of office divisions	4
Division of Preventive Medicine, 1940-44	4
Administrative Division, 1943-46	4
Field records	5
Case files for patients at naval hospitals and registers thereto, 1812-1944	5
Other field records, 1844-1920	5

INTRODUCTION

After the issuance of a preliminary inventory, it is sometimes necessary to bring the information up to date before further study can be made. Dates or quantities of records may need to be corrected, or entries for additional series may need to be inserted. This supplement to Preliminary Inventory No. 6 has been prepared to take care of any such changes that should be made in the original issuance and needs to be used in conjunction with it.

Corrected entries bear the original entry numbers and are in numerical order. Each entry usually contains only the title, inclusive dates, and quantity of records; the specific changes are marked by underscoring. Changes of a purely editorial nature are not being made.

Additional entries bear entry numbers to which suffixes A, B, C, and so on have been added to indicate the most appropriate place in the original issuance for their insertion. Center and side headings from the original issuance are repeated when needed for guidance. Where necessary, additional headings are supplied.

The volume of records in this record group has been decreased to 1,093 cubic feet, compared with 9,000 cubic feet reported in the original issuance in 1948. The decrease is caused by the disposal or transfer of records described in entries 27, 28, 33, 34, 38 (partial), 39, 46, 50, 51 (partial), and 52. The records of the Bureau of Medicine and Surgery now in the National Archives cover the period 1842-1951.

RECORDS OF THE BUREAU OF MEDICINE AND SURGERY

HEADQUARTERS RECORDS

Correspondence, 1842-1951

GENERAL CORRESPONDENCE. Jan. 1926-Dec. 1951. 510 ft.   15
    Arranged in three chronological subseries (1926-41, 1942-46, and 1947-51) according to the classification scheme of the Navy Filing Manual.

INDEX TO GENERAL CORRESPONDENCE. Jan. 1926-Dec. 1951. 35 ft.   22
    Arranged in three chronological subseries: 1926-41, 1942-46, and 1947-51.

Medical Journals and Reports on Patients, 1812-1940

MEDICAL JOURNALS OF SHORE STATIONS. 1812-89; 1911-15. 324 vols. 50 ft.   21

Medical Certificates and Casualty Lists, 1828-1939

MISCELLANEOUS RECORDS RELATING TO CASUALTY LISTS. 1861-1939. 1 in.   36A
    Arranged chronologically.

Sanitary and Other Reports, 1907-45

ANNUAL SANITARY REPORTS. 1907, 1919, 1927, and 1943. 18 ft.   38

Personnel Records, 1824-1930

REGISTERS SHOWING INDIVIDUAL SERVICE OF MEDICAL OFFICERS OF THE U.S. NAVY AND OF THE NAVAL RESERVE FORCE. ca. 1820-1930. 15 vols. 3 ft.   40A
    Arranged in two subseries and thereunder chronologically by date of appointment of officer: (1) regular medical officers, ca. 1820-1930 (9 volumes); and (2) medical officers, Naval Reserve Force, 1893-1923 (6 volumes). The first volume of subseries 1 is arranged by name of officer. Name index in each volume.

COMPILED LIST OF NAMES OF SURGEON'S STEWARDS AND A LIST OF DOCUMENTS CONCERNING THEM. 1 item.   45A
    Names are listed alphabetically; documents are listed numerically (and roughly chronologically) as they appear in the volumes described in entry 45.

Fiscal Records, 1854-1926

REQUISITIONS SENT TO THE SECRETARY OF THE NAVY REQUESTING FUNDS FOR NAVY AGENTS. Jan. 5, 1854-July 30, 1857. 2 vols. 3 in.
Arranged chronologically by year and thereunder numbered.   47A

JOURNAL OF EXPENDITURES ("DAY BOOK" AND "JOURNAL LETTER NO.5"). 1884-93, 1922-26. 2 vols. 2 ft.   48

Records Relating to the History of Naval Medicine, 1775-1946

RECORDS RELATING TO THE HISTORY OF NAVAL MEDICINE. 1775-1945. 6 ft.
Arranged according to a numerical classification scheme. A copy of the filing scheme is at the beginning of the series.   48A

HISTORICAL SUPPLEMENTS SUBMITTED WITH SANITARY REPORTS. 1941-46. 7 ft.
Arranged alphabetically by name of ship or station in two chronological subseries: (1) 1941-43 and (2) 1941-46.   48B

HISTORY OF THE NAVAL MEDICAL DEPARTMENT. 1941-45. 3 vols. 6 in.   48C
Arranged by subject. Each volume has a table of contents. Most of the volumes that were once part of this series are missing.

Records of Office Divisions

Division of Preventive Medicine, 1940-44

SECURITY-CLASSIFIED MINUTES, PUBLICATIONS, REPORTS, AND CORRESPONDENCE OF SUBCOMMITTEES OF THE DIVISION OF MEDICAL SCIENCE OF THE NATIONAL RESEARCH COUNCIL. 1940-43. 7 ft.   49A
Arranged by name of subcommittee or subject.

SECURITY-CLASSIFIED REPORTS OF COMMITTEES WORKING UNDER THE DIVISION OF MEDICAL SCIENCES OF THE NATIONAL RESEARCH COUNCIL AND THE OFFICE OF SCIENTIFIC RESEARCH AND DEVELOPMENT. 1940-44. 4 ft.   49B
Arranged by subject.

Administrative Division, 1943-46

CORRESPONDENCE, MEMORANDA, REPORTS, AND ISSUANCES OF THE ADMINISTRATIVE HISTORY SECTION. Dec. 1943-Feb. 1946. 4 in.   49C
Arranged chronologically.

FIELD RECORDS

Case Files for Patients at Naval Hospitals and Registers Thereto, 1812-1944

REGISTERS OF PATIENTS. 1812-1889. 38 vols. 12 ft.

Other Field Records, 1812-1846

LETTERS SENT BY THE U.S. NAVAL HOSPITAL, PORTSMOUTH, N.H., TO
THE SURGEON GENERAL OF THE NAVY. Mar. 1842-Aug. 1884. 1 vol.
1 in.
   Arranged chronologically. Subject index.

EXPENDITURE BOOK KEPT ON BOARD THE U.S. FRIGATE THE CLARIO
   BY SURGEON NINIAN PINKNEY. 1844-46. 1 vol. 1/2 in.
   Entries arranged by type of medical or hospital stores purchased.

www.ingramcontent.com/pod-product-compliance
Lightning Source LLC
Chambersburg PA
CBHW081351040426
42450CB00015B/3401